How to Go on a Diabetic Diet

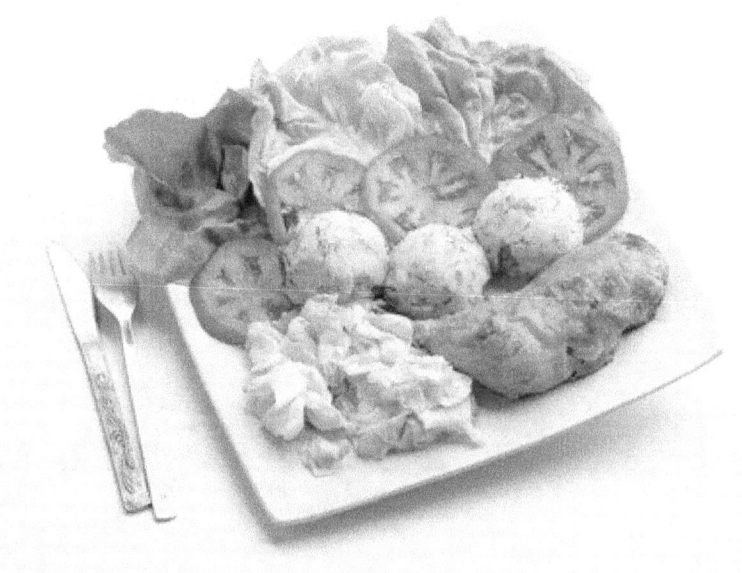

Lifestyle Changes That Put You Back in Control

Disclaimer

Although the author and publisher have made every effort to ensure that the information in this book was correct at press time, the author and publisher do not assume and hereby disclaim any liability to any party for any loss, damage, or disruption caused by errors or omissions, whether such errors or omissions result from negligence, accident, or any other cause.

Other Titles By This Author Include:

<u>Waistline Weight Loss Secrets To Getting A Flat Belly Fast: Imagine A Sexy You In 27 Days Or Less</u>

<u>Sweet Potato Recipes: Top 37 Easy, Quick, Healthy & Delicious Sweet Potato Recipes</u>

<u>The Power of Yoga and Meditation: The Ultimate Guide to a Peaceful Mental and Physical State with Yoga and Meditation</u>

<u>Vitamins and Supplements: Everything You Need to Know to Manage Your Own Health</u>

Grab The Entire Collection Today!

Table of contents

Introduction

Discovering you have diabetes or a problem with your blood sugar can be detrimental emotionally and physically. While your body physically struggles with the disease, emotionally you become bereft for all the things you are told you can no longer have to eat or drink. However, it does not have to be so dreary! You can go on a diabetic diet and enjoy it. You just have to know what your alternatives are.

There are many things that a person with diabetes or who is at risk for diabetes should not have. Chocolate, sweets like cakes and ice cream, pizza, and other foods that many of us take for granted. There are many beverages that should also be avoided, such as soft drinks and alcohol. However, there are generally alternatives to these foods and drinks that are just as yummy. You just have to give them a chance.

This short e-book will give you a start on planning your diabetic diet. It will give you tips and tricks for creating a diet you can live with. You will also learn about different aspects of a diabetes diet, and how it applies to life in general.

The goal here is to educate you as much as possible about how to plan, implement and stick to the lifestyle changes that are required for your continued good health. To determine the exact lifestyle changes you need to make and to create an actual diabetic diet plan, you should consult with your doctor or nutritionist for more information and details about what is right for you and your health plan.

Overall, you will learn about lifestyle changes that will greatly improve your blood sugar. It is entirely possible to manage diabetes with diet alone in many cases. If nothing else, sticking to a diabetic diet will enable you to take lower doses of insulin or medications. You just have to be determined that you are going to become a healthier you.

Creating a Diabetic Diet Plan

The first thing anyone wants to know is how to create a diabetic diet plan. You can purchase diet plans, but these are often difficult to stick to because they give you specific foods that you may or may not enjoy. Creating your own diabetic diet plan gives you the flexibility to include foods and meals that you will enjoy so that you can stick to your diet.

You can get help creating a diet plan from a nutritionist or your doctor. However, it is entirely possible to develop the plan on your own. However, you will want to run your plan by your doctor or nutritionist before putting it into effect. This way you can be certain that the plan you have come up with will actually be successful in controlling your blood sugar.

Getting Started

The first thing you have to do is educate yourself about what foods increase your blood sugar and decrease your health. There are obvious foods that will increase your blood sugar such as cookies, cakes, and other baked goods. It stands to reason that anything containing sugar is going to raise your blood sugar, and therefore should be avoided.

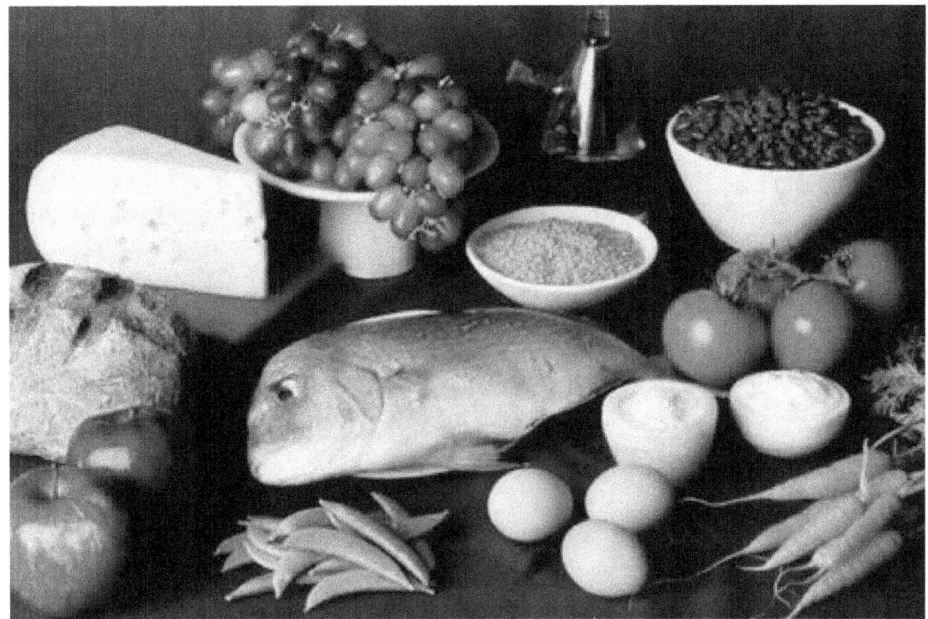

But there are many other foods that raise blood sugar. The most common of these are foods containing carbohydrates. Carbohydrates turn into blood glucose. This includes simple carbohydrates such as those found in fruits and vegetables, as well as complex carbohydrates such as those found in starches like pasta and potatoes.

It is these foods that you need to regulate in your diet plan and ensure you do not get too many of them. Your doctor or dietician can give you a better idea of how many carbohydrates you can take in each day or each meal and keep your blood sugar in check. This number can be different for everyone, based on weight, weight loss goals, and how drastic your blood sugar problem has become. However, you should keep in mind that cutting out carbohydrates altogether is not an option. You need carbohydrates in your diet to give you energy and keep your blood sugar from getting too low.

In addition to your blood sugar, you need to think about a heart healthy diet. Having diabetes or blood sugar problems increases your risk for heart disease and stroke. Therefore, there are other foods you should avoid in your diet plan. These include foods that contain saturated fats, Trans fats, cholesterol or sodium.

Keep in mind also when developing your diabetic diet plan that quality is more important than quantity when it comes to a diabetic diet. This means that how much you eat isn't as important as what you eat. If you struggle with hunger on a 2,000 calorie diet, try a 2,500 or 3,000 calorie diet. Just be sure that most of those calories are coming from foods that do not adversely affect your blood sugar or heart health.

Your diabetic diet plan should incorporate foods from all of the food groups to ensure you are getting all of the nutrients necessary for good health. You should make sure that you have certain nutrients in moderation rather than cutting them out altogether. In addition to various vitamins and minerals, you should ensure you are getting the following nutrients in healthy amounts.

- Proteins are important for cell growth and maintenance

- Good fats such as polyunsaturated and monounsaturated fats are important for healthy cells

- Sodium in moderate amounts is required for good health

- Fiber is an important part of digestive health

Typical Daily Allowances for Diabetics

It is important that you look at your whole health when developing your diabetic diet. To that end, you should take into consideration the daily allowances of different food groups that you should have each day. This will help you plan your diet.

- 2 servings of meat

- 2 servings of dairy

- 3 servings of fruits

- 4 servings of vegetables

- 8 servings of whole grains

- Up to 4 good fats like olive oil or real butter

Making a List of Foods

With all of these facts in mind, you are ready to start actually planning your diabetic diet. Start your plan by making a list of foods that are acceptable and a list of foods that are unacceptable. On your list of foods that are acceptable, you should have plenty of fruits and vegetables, lean meats, and whole grains.

Do not just come up with a list of acceptable foods by surfing the internet and writing down every food that is good for you. Instead, use these online food lists as a source of ideas. Write down on your list only those foods that you know you will enjoy eating. There is no need to detest your diet plan by putting foods on the menu that you know you don't like.

Be sure to include several things on your list. You need to have the food, the appropriate serving size, the total grams of fat, and the total grams of carbohydrates. You may also want to include the total grams of sodium, cholesterol, and protein. You will need all of this information when you start creating meals for your diet plan.

Next, make a list of foods that you enjoy but should not be a part of your diet plan. This may seem a bit depressing, but there is good reason for it. Not only will it keep you from putting those foods into your diet plan, it will also give you a list to work from for substitutions.

Go through your list of foods that you cannot include in your diet plan and search the internet for substitutions. If you really like pasta you can substitute whole wheat pasta for the starchier counterpart. If you really like chocolate or baked goods containing chocolate, look for recipes and pre-made goodies made with sugar substitute and carob chips or cocoa.

The possible substitutions are nearly endless. Put these substitutions on your list of foods to include in your meal plan. Don't forget serving size. This is very important when it comes to substitutions as well as typical foods.

Finally, start a list of foods that are great for your health but you have never tried before. These foods can be slowly introduced into your diet plan, and if you do not like them you can remove them from the plan later. This gives you more choices in your meal planning.

To expand your lists, hit the grocery store for some browsing. Check out the nutrition labels on some of your favorite foods to see which list they belong on. Check out foods as well that you have never tried before. This is especially helpful if you like to eat prepared foods or dinners that you heat and eat.

You can put those meals on your list of acceptable foods if they are within the limits of your ideal carbohydrate count. If they aren't, add them to your list of unacceptable foods. You may be able to develop a recipe to recreate the dish in a lower carbohydrate form.

You should also check out the health food section of your store. There is usually a diabetic section in the bakery that offers sugar free foods, as well as a sugar free section in the candy aisle. Other diabetic foods may be offered in the health foods or whole foods section of the store. This can give you further ideas for your meal options.

Coming Up with Meal Options

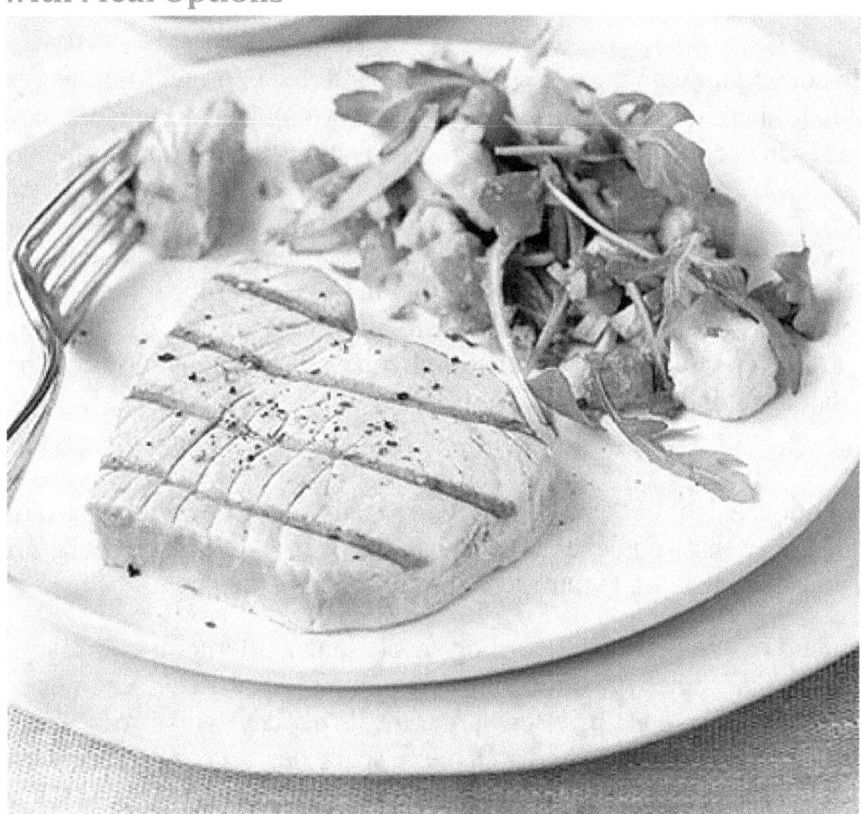

Your next step in creating a diabetic diet is to come up with meals that you can use in your diet plan. You should have a large variety of meals for breakfast, lunch and dinner. You should also make sure you come up with many snack options. These meals should take into account the number of carbohydrates you should have at each time of day. Again, a dietician or your doctor can assist you in knowing how many carbohydrates you need throughout the day, and when you should have them.

Make your own meal options by combining foods from your appropriate foods list. Keep in mind the recommended serving sizes when creating these meals, as well as the appropriate number of grams of carbohydrates, fat and protein. Your meals should be well rounded, giving you a variety of nutrients throughout the day. Your meals should include the following components.

Breakfast, Lunch and Dinner:

- Protein such as a lean meat, eggs, beans or peanut butter

- Whole grain such as bread, oatmeal, or pasta

- Vegetables or fruits should be 2/3 of your plate

- Dairy such as a glass of milk, a piece of cheese, or a cup of yogurt

Fruits and vegetables should comprise the largest part of your morning and afternoon snacks. You may also want to include a dairy item with your snacks such as a glass of milk or a cup of yogurt in the evenings. The dairy will help fill you up, and the calcium is important for good bone health.

If you need help coming up with meal options, hit the internet. You will find many sample menus that will help spark ideas. The meals in these menus may be acceptable to you as they are. Alternatively, you can use them as a starting point substituting foods on your personal acceptable list for those foods you don't particularly like.

If you aren't very creative in coming up with meals, or if you prefer one dish meals, you can find a wealth of resources for diabetic recipes on the internet or at your local library. There are a plethora of diabetic cookbooks available from many different sources. Don't be afraid to try new things. However, to keep your diet plan something you can live with you should primarily choose recipes that contain the foods on your personal acceptable food list.

The Menu

When you have completed all of these steps you are ready to start developing your menu or meal plan. It is recommended that you develop your plan one week at a time. Use the information you have gathered, your food lists, and your meal options to create the menu.

Each day you should have a breakfast, morning snack, lunch, afternoon snack, and dinner. You may also want to include some type of dessert or evening snack as well. Eating several small meals each day is preferable to eating a few larger meals per day. This is especially true when developing a diabetic diet plan, because you have to space out your carbohydrates and sugars to ensure that you do not experience a spike or plummet in your blood sugar. At the same time you need a certain amount of carbohydrates in order to have the energy you need throughout the day. Therefore it is important to spread out those carbohydrates in small meals. This will also keep you from eating too much, or feeling too hungry throughout the day.

What to Avoid When Creating Your Diet Plan

There are certain things that you should avoid when creating your diet plan. Incorporating these things into your diet plan by avoiding the pitfalls is important for overall dietary success in controlling your diabetes and becoming less dependent on medication. Start with these basics.

- Don't combine diets because they look good on paper. Either create your own diet from scratch or choose one particular diet from the internet or a reference book. But do not combine or alter diets found online or in reference materials. You will make a mistake and you will damage your chances of success.

- Don't forget to go lean on all of your dietary choices. Just because you can eat meat doesn't mean to pick the juiciest, fattest cut. Just because you can eat grilled chicken doesn't mean you smother it in fattening sauces. And, a salad benefits you nothing if covered in fatty dressing.

- Don't take the night off to dine out. Make wise choices when eating out just as you would when you are eating in. Make sure you only eat the appropriate serving size, and not try to eat everything on your plate.

- Don't leave out physical activity. Getting good exercise is an important part of a diabetic diet. It is scientifically proven that exercise and diet together can treat type 2 diabetes without the need for medication or insulin. Don't undermine yourself by forgetting this important step.

Gluten Free and Diabetic Diet Foods

Sometimes it is difficult to know which foods to include in your diabetic diet plan. After all, there are other considerations to be made for your diet other than just being sugar free and low carb. Here are some helpful tips on gluten free and diabetic diet foods.

Why Gluten Free?

If you are experiencing gluten intolerance or you have celiac disease, you should also include foods in your diabetic diet that are gluten free. Gluten is a protein found in certain whole grains such as wheat, rye, and barley. When you go gluten free, it is necessary to include alternative whole grains into your diet.

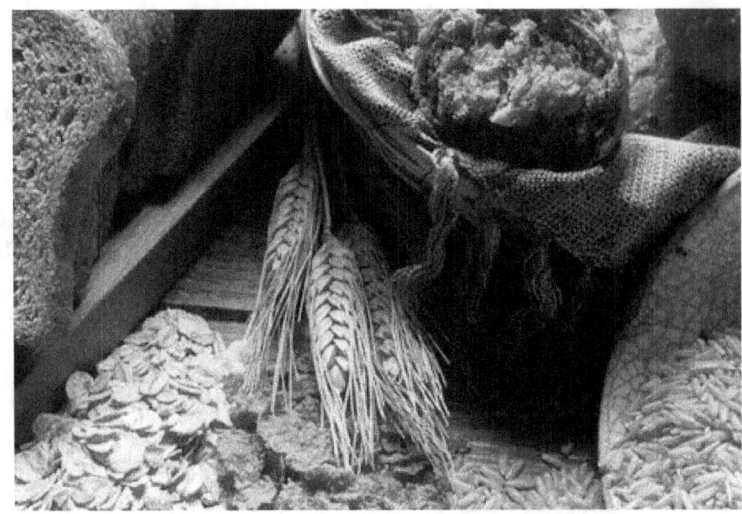

Gluten intolerance usually presents itself as pain in the abdomen when you eat foods loaded with gluten. Celiac disease causes damage to your small intestine when you eat gluten, and is present in about ten percent of patients with type 1 diabetes. If you have questions about whether or not to include gluten free foods in your diabetic diet, check with your doctor or nutritionist.

A Cautionary Note

Diabetic diet foods are good for you because they are developed specifically to work with a diabetic diet. However, it is vital that you remember that serving size is key to making the diabetic diet work to control your blood sugar. Even if you are eating diabetic diet foods, you can still manage to have a blood sugar spike or drop if you eat too much.

Therefore, in any type of diet, portion size is important. If a serving of pasta is one third of a cup, you should only eat that one serving of pasta. Have some sides of vegetables and include some pieces of a lean meat to flesh it out and make it more of a meal.

The following lists of gluten free and diabetic diet foods will help you add to your possible menu options for your diabetic diet. This list is in no way comprehensive. There are many foods out there, too many to list in one short e-book.

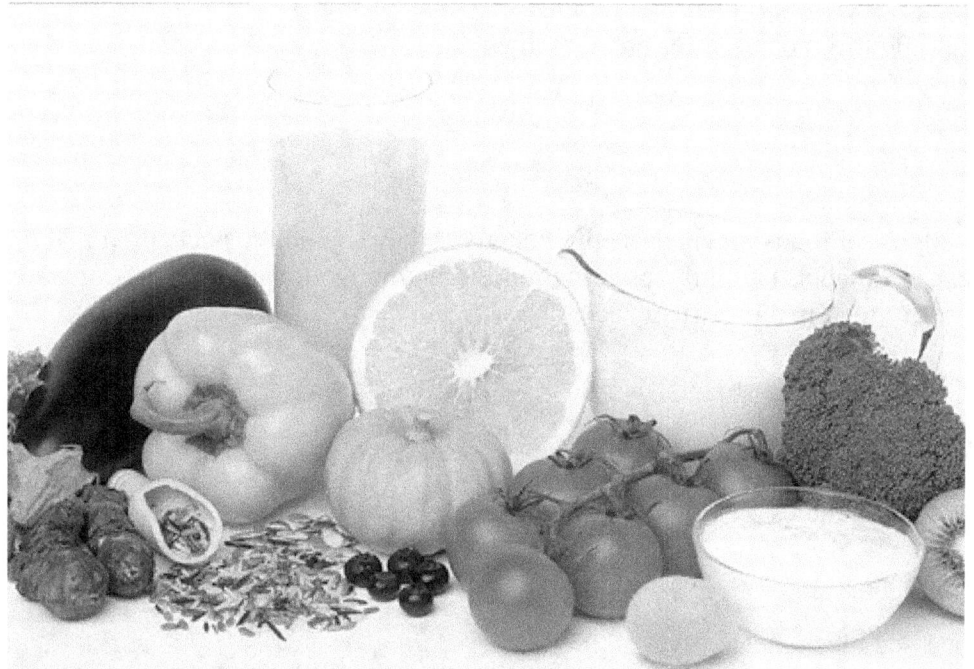

In most cases, there is a gluten free alternative or substitute for the foods you enjoy that have gluten in them. For example, you can make baked goods with rice flour instead of white flour. The easiest way to look for gluten free foods is to hit your local health food store and stroll down the gluten free aisle. However, there are some foods that are naturally gluten free that can be included in your diet.

The following list of foods is acceptable on a gluten free and diabetic diet.

- Beans

- Seeds

- Nuts

- Eggs

- Lean meats, fish and poultry with no breading, batter coating, or marinade

- Fruits

- Vegetables

- Most dairy products

- Buckwheat flour and products can be substituted

- Corn and cornmeal can be substituted for some recipes

- Flax meal

- Rice flour can be substituted in many baked goods recipes

- Potato flour can be used for bread recipes

- Rice

- Soy

The following list of foods may be acceptable only if they say on the packaging that they are gluten free. Check labels carefully, as some foods that you would not think of containing gluten are actually very high in the nutrient.

- Breads

- Sugar free baked goods

- Sugar free candies

- Gravies

- Processed lunch meats

- French fries

- Soups and soup bases

- Salad dressings

- Frozen vegetables in sauce

- All sauces

- Seasoned rice mixes

- Cereals

- Pastas

Again, this list is in no way exhaustive. However, it does present a list of foods that are both gluten free and sugar free and therefore friendly to your diabetic diet plan.

Diabetic Diet Foods

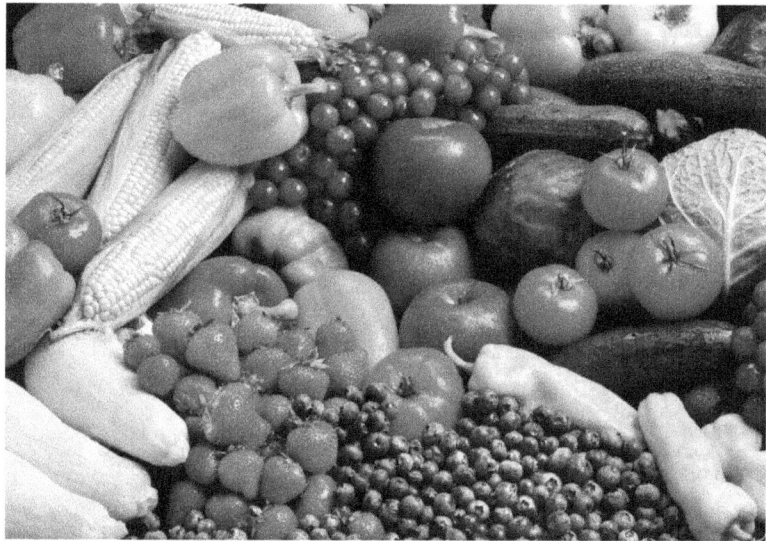

Diabetic diet foods are also important. It is important to choose foods that are completely sugar free. It is also important to choose foods with a low glycemic index. Foods with a low glycemic index have few carbohydrates, or carbohydrates that do not induce blood sugar spikes. They tend to fill you up longer, and keep your blood sugar regulated.

If you are curious about the glycemic index of any given food, you can easily look it up at GlycemicIndex.com. A food with a glycemic index of over seventy is considered high and should be avoided or limited. However, the following list of foods will help you stick to a diabetic diet with low glycemic index foods that are also gluten free.

- Green leafy vegetables

- Squash

- Asparagus

- Okra, not battered and fried

- Pickles and cucumbers

- Brussels sprouts

- Eggplant

- Onions

- Tomatoes

- Cauliflower and broccoli

- Peas

- Buckwheat bread

- Corn or corn meal

- Most fruits

- Sweet potatoes and potatoes

- Beans

- Yogurt

The Best Type of Diet for a Diabetic

The best type of diet for a diabetic will be determined by that individual's personal health. There is no magic diet plan that works for all diabetics. Each individual is different. Each individual has their own tastes and cravings, and those must be taken into account also when developing the diabetic diet.

However, there are some basic guidelines that all diabetics should follow in order to control their blood sugar. You will need to count carbohydrates, fats, proteins, and cholesterol for a wholly healthy diet.

Counting Carbohydrates

You should concentrate on counting carbohydrates. Carbohydrates will bump up your blood sugar faster than any other type of food. It is only by counting carbohydrates that you can manage your blood sugar. There are three ways that you can do this.

The Exchange Diet

One type of diabetic diet uses exchanges. With exchanges, foods are placed into groups of foods with like amounts of carbohydrates. You then choose a food from that group for your menu. For example, if your meal plan says you can have an apple, you can exchange that apple for a third cup of pasta while dining out.

Exchanges work well for many people because they know exactly what they can have. It is easier to keep track of a few food choices in each group than to manually count carbohydrates. It is also easier than trying to determine the glycemic index of foods. You can find many exchange type diabetic diets online, in your local library, or by visiting your nutritionist or doctor.

Exchanges have another benefit. You can easily enjoy some of the foods you might otherwise be missing as long as you take them in moderation. You can exchange a piece of fruit for a handful of potato chips. It may not be the best thing for your health, and you should not do it all the time, but it is an option. Exchanges offer you that flexibility.

Manually Counting Carbs

Finally, you can do a more complicated diabetic diet in which you actually manually count the carbohydrates that you take in each meal. You will need to space out your carbohydrate intake throughout the day so that you have the energy you need without causing a spike in your blood sugar. This is the type of diet outlined in the first section of this e-book. It offers the most flexibility in the foods you eat, but takes the most time to put into effect.

The Glycemic Index Diet

The second type of diabetic diet is where you base your food choices on the glycemic index. In order to do this you will need a good resource and the time to research the foods that you want to include in your diet plan. There are many websites available to help you do this absolutely free; you just have to have the time to do the research. By eating foods with a glycemic index of sixty or lower, you will be able to effectively manage your blood sugar.

For most diabetics, this is not an option. Judging your foods only by the glycemic index without counting carbohydrates can lead to consuming more carbohydrates than you should have in one meal. While foods with a low glycemic index are indeed healthier for diabetics, eating too much of one food or too many of a combination of foods can lead to a blood sugar spike.

The Differences in Diabetes Diets

The biggest difference in diabetes diets is what type of diabetes you are treating. If you are treating Type 1 diabetes, you will need to have a different and more structured diet than if you are treating Type 2 diabetes. The same is true for juvenile diabetes. Here are some basic guidelines on the different types of diets.

Type 1 Diabetes Diets

When you have Type 1 diabetes you are likely managing your diabetes with the use of routine insulin. This fact makes it very important that you eat the same amount of carbohydrates at the same times every day. This allows for an extremely structured diet.

Manually counting carbohydrates works best for this type of diet. You want to be certain you are getting the exact same amount of carbohydrates at each meal each day. This is important for the insulin to work properly and keep your blood sugar at optimum levels.

Type 2 Diabetes Diets

Type 2 diabetes diets can be less structured. The purpose of these diets is to keep the blood sugar from spiking by controlling the amount of carbohydrates you take in throughout each day. This type of diet is the most common and often considered diabetes diet in America.

Exchange diets work well for this type of diabetes. The exact number of carbohydrates need not be consistent with each meal of each day. It matters only that you do not exceed the recommended amount of carbohydrates. It is also important that you spread out your carbohydrates throughout the day so that you do not experience a blood sugar spike.

Juvenile Diabetes

Juvenile diabetes is actually the same thing as Type 1 diabetes. However, in children and teenagers it is even more important to have a structured diet. Children and teens with juvenile diabetes should have their carbohydrates carefully counted and planned by their parents. They should only take packed lunches to school and not eat cafeteria lunches. They should also be very careful about what they eat at friend's homes or parties.

Gestational Diabetes Diets

Gestational diabetes is when you develop high blood sugar levels while pregnant. Managing this type of diet can be difficult. You must be sure that you are not eating anything that will raise your blood sugar too high, while also making sure you are getting enough nutrients for both you and your baby. A nutritionist can better help you develop a diabetes diet for this situation, as each mother is different and the guidelines for these types of diets are much different from other types of diabetes.

Keeping it Heart Healthy

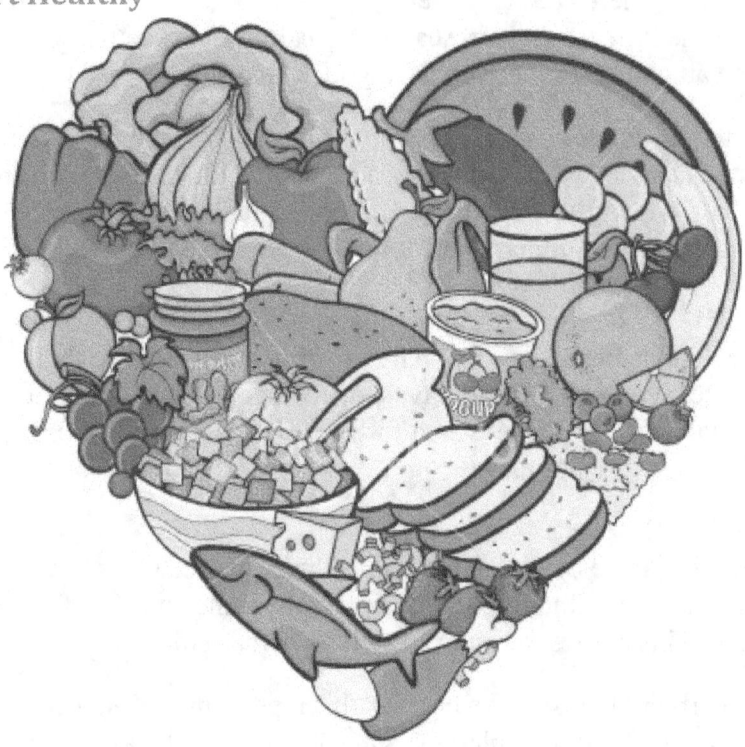

Since diabetics are more likely to be at risk for heart disease and stroke, it is important to also have a heart healthy diet. This means that you need to watch your fat and cholesterol intake. You should also be watching your sodium intake. At the same time, you want to be certain you are getting the proteins you need for a healthy lifestyle.

This may seem like a lot to track, but it becomes easier as you get used to it. If you keep in mind all of these aspects of your diabetic diet, you will be able to easily create meal options and menu plans for yourself with little difficulty. In fact, over time it will become second nature, and you will not have to think about it much at all.

The following foods are best for a heart healthy diet:

- Lean meats that are grilled or baked without breading or marinade

- Good fats such as olive oil

- Low sodium foods and sodium free seasonings

- Beans, lentils, and other legumes for protein with good fats

- Fish with important Omega 3 Fatty Acids

Who Benefits from a Diabetic Diet

A diabetic diet is not just for people with diabetes. Those who have a high risk of diabetes or other blood sugar problems that can lead to diabetes may be told to go on a diabetic diet by their doctor. However, the question often arises of whether or not a diabetic diet is safe for everyone.

The fact of the matter is that most people can benefit from a diabetic diet. The diabetic diet is full of vegetables and fruits, with little sweet treats and only the amount of meats and dairy required for good health. Everyone should be eating a heart healthy diet, and cutting the sugar and carbohydrates down in your diet can go a long ways toward increasing your health and lifestyle.

The following people should definitely consider a diabetic diet:

- Those who have a direct relative with Type 2 diabetes, such as mother or grandparent
- Those who are overweight
- Those who tend to have high blood sugar, although it may be within the higher ranges of normal levels
- Those who tend to have low blood sugar, but within normal levels
- Those who have experienced gestational diabetes
- Those with high blood pressure (over 140/90)
- Those with a sedentary lifestyle, meaning that you do not have much physical activity
- Those in the higher age bracket, usually 45 or older

In fact, most people benefit right away from the diabetic diet. By ditching sugars and counting carbohydrates, many people find that they lose weight rather quickly, and they are able to keep that weight off by continuing their healthy dietary eating habits. In addition, people on a diabetic diet decrease their risk of diabetes, heart disease, and other health conditions.

If everyone ate a diabetic diet, the nation would be in a much healthier state than it is in today. The number of obese people would decrease, the number of cases of heart disease and stroke would decrease, and the number of people with diabetes would decrease. If you are considering a diabetic diet for any reason, take the plunge. You will not regret it.

How to Implement a Diabetic Diet

Implementing a diabetic diet can be much more difficult that planning it. It can be a very hard thing to give up the foods you have been eating possibly for your entire life. It can be even harder to start and stick to a diet plan that includes foods you normally don't eat. Here are some tips for implementing a diabetic diet you can stick with.

General Tips for Success

These basic tips will help you be successful in your diabetic diet. By making these simple, small lifestyle changes, you will discover that you are able to manage your diabetes with diet easily.

- Watch your serving sizes. This is most important when it comes to meat, fruit and grains. It is very easy to overeat with these foods. Make sure you are only eating the appropriate number of servings a day and not the huge portions Americans are used to eating.

- Chew your food slowly. Put down your fork between bites. Take a drink of water every few bites. All of these actions will help prevent you from overeating.

- Start an exercise routine. Even if you just walk a few blocks each evening, you are doing some type of physical activity. This is important to support your diabetic diet.

- Don't try to eat the same thing every week. You will quickly get tired of your diet and want to make a change, usually for the worse. Have lots of meal options available to you so that you can change it up every week and not become bored.

- Switch to eating as many fresh and organic foods as possible. This will not only improve your health, but it will naturally cut down on the amounts of sodium, bad fats, cholesterol, and carbohydrates you take in each day.

Will Power and Determination

However, it is important that you implement your diabetic diet as quickly as possible to gain control over your blood sugar. You will need to stick to your diet as closely as possible in order to maintain good health. While this is easier said than done, it is possible if you have the mentality necessary to make it happen.

Starting a new diet and making lifestyle changes is never easy. It requires a certain amount of will power and determination. You have to put it into your mind that you are ready to tackle these lifestyle changes.

Motivation

It is also important to keep yourself motivated to start the diet and maintain it. Obviously, your health is a great motivator. However, sometimes this is not enough to motivate you to keep yourself from eating that piece of chocolate cake for dessert. You have to come up with other motivators.

One trick that is often used by weight loss dieters is to purchase a dress or outfit in your goal size and hang it on your bedroom wall. This serves as a standing reminder of what you are working towards. The same type of motivation can be had for a diabetic diet, but somewhat in reverse.

If you are trying to stay independent of insulin by controlling your blood sugar with diet, post a picture of an insulin shot or something similar on your refrigerator. It will help you keep in mind what you are working toward, or rather away from. With this constant unpleasant reminder, you should be able to resist that piece of chocolate cake.

There are other ways to motivate yourself as well. You can reward yourself with sugar free sweets on weekends when you have stuck to your diet all week long. If you don't stick to your diet, you don't get the sweets at the end of the week. It is kind of the same principle as rewarding children for good behavior. You know that if you stick to your diet you will have something to look forward to, and that is great motivation if you can stick to your guns about it.

Another great motivator is to be held accountable for your diet by others. If you are married, make your spouse hold you accountable for your eating habits and sticking to your diabetic diet. If you are not married, find a good friend or family member to do this for you. This individual should be the person you go to whenever you feel like cheating on your diabetic diet. It should also be someone you talk to daily so that they can ask how you are doing on implementing your diet, holding you accountable to someone.

Taking it One Step at a Time

If possible, you should make lifestyle changes slowly. Take things one step at a time. Concentrate on cutting sugar out of your diet first, and then worry about counting carbohydrates. Once you have that down you can start working on the heart healthy part of your diet plan. Trying to switch your eating habits immediately and without preamble can make implementing the diet that much more difficult.

Of course, there are situations in which the change must be made immediately for your health. If this is the case, you should change your eating habits right away and as much as possible. The first step in this case is to empty the house of any foods that are not on your diabetic diet plan. You should also refrain from eating out for a period of time. At that point, you will be doing well if you can avoid purchasing any of those foods that you are not supposed to be eating.

Diabetic Diet Plans for Travelers

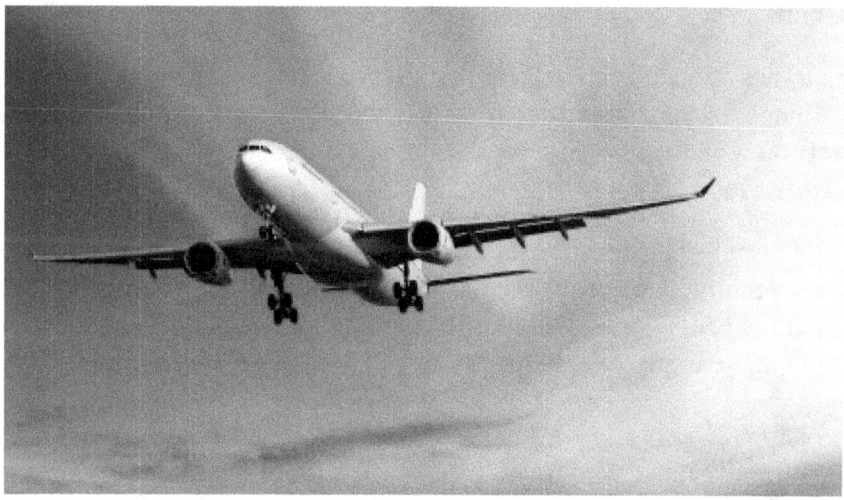

Going on any diet when you are traveling can be really difficult. Starting a diabetic diet when you are always on the road or in the air can be extremely difficult. When you are traveling a lot, you tend to eat out more than you cook for yourself. This is understandable. However, it is important to keep in mind your dietary concerns when eating out.

The best diabetic plan for travelers is to count carbohydrates. This requires you to have a reference book that will outline for you the carbohydrate content of common foods. This way you can check foods against the book to count your carbohydrates for each meal you eat while you are on the road.

Exchanges do not work well for travelers because your food options may be limited. In addition, it is not always possible to know the glycemic index for foods offered by restaurants. However, most fast food restaurants have nutritional information available for their menu items that includes carbohydrate counts. Therefore, manually counting your carbohydrates is generally the way to go in this situation.

Restaurants

The important thing to remember about restaurants is that their portion sizes are way out of control. Most restaurants serve up a piece of meat that is the equivalent of two or three servings. The same is true of side dishes, usually with the exception of vegetables.

To eliminate problems with your blood sugar and to maintain a heart healthy diet, you will want to be careful about what you order at restaurants. You will want to avoid any foods that are fried or breaded in any way. Grilled foods are best, and are available at nearly any restaurant. You can then cut the meat into two or three portions, eat one portion and take the rest with you to the hotel for a quick meal later in the day or the next day. Most hotel rooms have microwaves for this purpose.

You also need to watch what sides you order. Avoid starchy foods such as baked potatoes and French fries. Instead, order lots of vegetables, and maybe a side of fruit. You will probably want to order sides in addition to the ones available for your entrée. This is due to the fact that vegetable portions are typically small in restaurants, and you want two thirds of your meal to be fruits and vegetables.

The type of restaurant you visit is also important. Stay away from Italian restaurants, as pasta is one of the worst things for your blood sugar and the portions served up by these restaurants is way out of proportion with the amount you should be eating. The best type of restaurant to eat in is a buffet with lots of food choices.

Buffets tend to have smaller pieces of meat available making it easier to control your serving sizes. You also have complete control over the size of your portions of vegetables and fruits, and you can have as many vegetables as you like with most diabetic diets. Buffets do not allow for leftovers and can be more expensive, but it is worth it to stay on your diabetic diet.

Fast Food

Many travelers, especially those who travel by car, eat a lot of fast food. You can safely do this if you do it right. You have to be very careful about what you are ordering. You do not want any foods that are fried or breaded. Again, grilled is best. Most fast food restaurants have grilled options.

However, choosing a grilled chicken sandwich is not necessarily the way to go. If you order it as generally made, it will come loaded with fatty mayonnaise. Additionally, the bread in the bun is much more than you should have for carbohydrates for a meal as a diabetic. To fix this, order your grilled chicken sandwich plain, and eat it without the bun. For some added flavor, you can ask for some fat free ranch dressing to top the chicken.

Sides are also a problem with fast food restaurants. French fries, especially those from fast food restaurants, will cause your blood sugar to spike dangerously. Most fast food restaurants allow you to substitute a side salad for the French fries. You can also order a yogurt parfait to get in a fruit and some dairy into your meal.

Cooking Fresh is Always Best

Cooking your own meals is always the best option. When traveling it is generally possible to get a room with a mini fridge and a microwave. Some rooms come complete with kitchenettes. These features generally do not cost much more than rooms without them, and it is well worth the money to be able to maintain your diabetic diet while on the road. You can hit the grocery store locally to pick up the foods you need to stay on your diet. Microwaveable meals are often acceptable if you choose the right ones. As always, watch food labels.

Diabetes Diets for Preventing Diabetes

Many people who have a high risk for developing diabetes want to know if a diabetic diet can help prevent them from getting diabetes later on down the road. The answer to this question is not a simple one. It usually depends on the individual. However, there are some general answers that tend to be true for nearly everyone.

The fact of the matter is that if you are at high risk for diabetes, you need to be controlling your blood sugar now to avoid problems later. If you do develop diabetes later due to other complications or genetics, it will be much more possible to control your diabetes with diet if you have already adopted that type of lifestyle.

In the meantime, controlling your blood sugar with diet before getting diabetes can help lower your risk of developing the disease. It does not guarantee that you will not develop diabetes, but it does lower your risk. What this means is that the individual person may still develop diabetes, even if they take all of the precautions. The exact reason for this is not the same for everyone, and may not even be known. More research is being done all the time to determine why some people develop diabetes while others with the same risk factors do not.

The important thing to remember is that by lowering your risk, you are upping your chances of not dealing with the disease. If nothing else, going on the diabetic diet will make you healthier and help you lose weight. There is really no downside to going on a diabetic diet.

There are certain things you should do in addition to going on a diabetic diet if you are serious about preventing diabetes. These things will further decrease your risk of developing diabetes in the future. While diet is the most important, adding these things to your lifestyle will take you far in your quest for a healthier you.

- Get more exercise. The more exercise you get the lower your risk of diabetes. It is recommended that healthy adults get at least 300 minutes of aerobic exercise each week, and 100 minutes of strength training each week.

- Get more fiber in your diet. Fiber helps regulate your blood sugar, improves digestion, and promotes weight loss.

- Get more whole grains in your diet. Scientific evidence is still mounting on why, but it appears that increasing whole grains can decrease your risk of developing diabetes.

- Lose some weight. If you are overweight at all, you should look at ways to get down to your goal weight to further decrease your risk of diabetes. The diabetes diet and increased exercise alone will go a long way toward meeting this goal.

Diabetic Diets for Young Adults

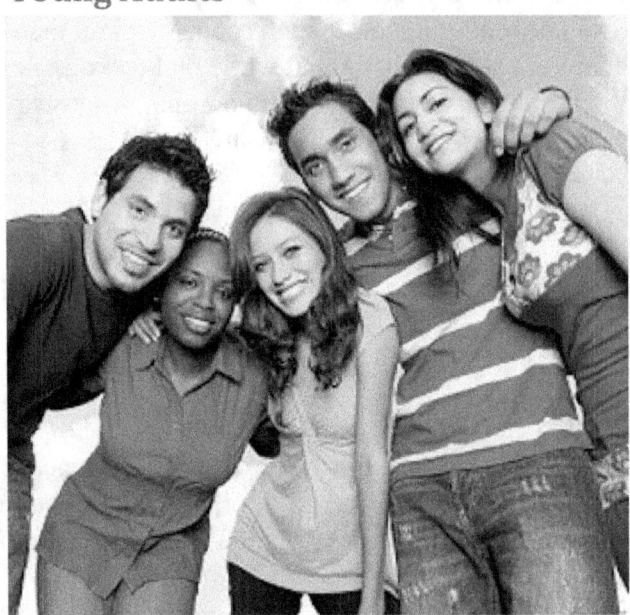

Diabetic diets for young adults should look much the same as a diabetic diet for older adults. The biggest difference is that young adults tend to burn more calories than older adults, and therefore need more calories in their diet. They also need the energy to burn those calories, which mean more carbohydrates in some cases.

However, on the other hand, diabetes in adults who developed the disorder at a younger age tend to have less success in managing their diabetes with diet and exercise alone. In order to avoid being one of these statistics, you should make sure that you take your diabetes in control now. That means losing weight and becoming healthy for a lifetime.

It is still important to keep carbohydrates to a minimum when you are on a diabetic diet. However, the minimum amount of carbohydrates for a young adult may be different than an adult in their mid life. Your doctor or nutritionist can give you a definitive response as to how many carbohydrates you should be getting and when throughout the day.

It is also important to note that the exchange diet works best for young adults. These individuals lead very busy lives, and do not necessarily want to take the time out to count carbohydrates. It is much easier for them to memorize the servings and groups of carbohydrates and make exchanges than to sit down and manually count their carbs.

Substitutions

The most important thing for young adults with a diabetic diet is to make sure that you have plenty of substitutions for the types of things young adults typically eat. As a young adult with diabetes, you will want to carry these substitute foods with you wherever you go, especially when you are hanging out with friends. While others are munching on candy and treats, you can enjoy some sugar free candy from your purse or backpack.

It is also a good idea to pack your lunch every day rather than depend on the food in the cafeteria at your job or college. This way you have more control over how you eat and what you eat, and you can still enjoy lunch with your friends. If someone offers you a food that you're not sure you should have, opt for something else that is available instead. Carrying fruit and other snacks with you is very helpful in this endeavor.

Everything in Moderation

Another thing to keep in mind as a young adult is that you can have certain things with your friends as long as you keep it in proportion. For example, if you are at a party where there is cake, you can have a very small one inch square of the cake to be polite and enjoy the flavor. If you are at the mall and everyone is getting pizza, you can too. Just be sure that you get thin crust and don't eat the extra bread without toppings. Keep toppings to veggies, with maybe one lean meat like chicken. You should also go light on the sauce.

In general, you can eat out with your friends as long as you maintain serving sizes and make wise food choices. The same rules that apply to travelers apply to anyone who is eating out on a regular basis. Take portion sizes into careful consideration, and make your choices of entrees and sides very carefully.

Eating Habits for a Lifetime

Remember that it is much easier to start a diabetic diet at this age than it is later on down the road. If you start your diabetic diet now, eventually you won't miss the foods you cannot have. As you get older you will need to change your diet slightly, but these changes will be minimal and have little effect on your quality of life.

In short, you are creating eating habits for a lifetime. Embrace your newly found lifestyle and do your best to support it faithfully. Having diabetes as a young adult can seem like an incredible pain, but really it is better to have to make those changes early on in life. In addition, making those changes now and managing your weight and diet now will help prevent you from having to become insulin dependent later in life.

Sticking to a Diabetic Plan

Implementing a diabetic diet plan may seem difficult enough in and of itself, but sticking to that diet plan can be excruciating. This is especially true if you have typically eaten a lot of sweets. How do you stay away from those foods that you know you shouldn't have, but that you crave so much?

Will Power and Determination

As mentioned earlier, implementing and sticking to a diabetic diet is largely a matter of will power and determination to do the right thing for your health. You must have the will to turn down those foods that are unhealthy for you. You must be determined enough to maintain a healthy lifestyle that you can turn down those sweets whenever they present themselves.

Removing Temptation

Your first step in making sure that you stick to your diabetic diet is to remove temptation. Don't go out to eat for a while until you are certain you can stick to your diet even when faced with unhealthy alternatives. Remove all unhealthy foods from your cabinets and refrigerator, getting rid of everything including the sugar.

This may upset the rest of your family, but it is necessary in order to stick to a diet. When faced with temptation in our weakest moments, we will always give in. It is human nature.

If you find yourself tempted into impulse buys while at the grocery store, have someone else do your shopping for you. Make a detailed grocery list based on your diabetic meal plan, and turn that list over to someone you can trust. Some grocery stores take your list and do the shopping for you, allowing you to then pick up your order without wandering the tempting aisles. Some stores will also deliver, allowing you to avoid the temptation of the store entirely.

Make Substitutions

Nearly any sweet treat that you are used to having has a sugar free counterpart. You can make sugar free baked goods yourself using diabetic recipes that make use of sugar substitutes such as Stevia, Splenda, Sweet and Low, Equal, or Sugar Twin. You can also substitute carob chips for chocolate. This way you can enjoy a piece of chocolate cake or some chocolate chip cookies without going off your diet.

You can also easily find sugar free versions of your favorite cookies and pies, as well as candy at your local grocery store. More and more people are being diagnosed with diabetes every day, and as a result the sugar free foods industry is booming. Nearly any grocery store in the nation has at least some sugar free foods throughout their store or in their bakery section.

The other thing you can do is retrain your brain to accept different types of sweetness to satisfy cravings. Instead of eating baked goods, eat a piece of fruit like an apple or banana. The sweetness of it is different, but it may be enough to satisfy your sweet tooth in a pinch.

Being Accountable

Being held accountable for your actions tends to make most people stick to what they are supposed to be doing. Obviously, your doctor is going to hold you accountable for your dietary habits. But often that is not enough for most people. The doctor is an outsider in your life, someone that can be easily ignored.

It is important to have someone in your life that holds you accountable for your eating habits. This person should check up on you, be there for you when you are tempted to go off your diet, and be willing to give you some tough love. Of course, you also have to be willing and able to take it for what it is.

This person in your life can be your spouse, child, or parent. If none of these apply to you, you can choose a good friend to be your back up when it comes to your diet. The person should be someone you trust, whose opinion matters to you greatly. It should also be someone nearby that can really ride you if necessary.

Being accountable for your actions should be enough to deter you from sneaking in that bowl of ice cream. It is not much fun or enjoyable to do something that you know you will get into trouble for later with someone you care about. However, sometimes even that is not enough.

Staying Motivated

We talked about motivation somewhat when discussing how to implement a diabetic diet plan. Now you will need to take this motivation one step further in order to stick to the diet plan you have put into place for yourself.

Find what motivates you to eat the way you should. Different people are motivated by different things. You have to take a hard look at yourself and decide what motivates you the most.

For some people, money is the only motivator for anything. Therefore, consider the money you will save on doctor's visits and medications by sticking to your diet. If you must, write these potential costs down and post it on your refrigerator.

If that is not enough for you, you can reward yourself with money or some other reward. Decide what your reward is going to be if you stick to your diet without cheating for just one month. It could be a small shopping spree, a new video game, or something else you've been wanting. When you accomplish your goal, reward yourself. Then, set a new goal.

Adjusting Naturally

Eventually you will no longer need any type of crutch or motivation to keep you on track. Once you become used to the lifestyle changes you are making, you will only think about those things you've been missing every once in a great long while. When you do think about them, it will just be a passing thought.

Planning a Diabetic Diet for a Young Picky Eater

Planning a diabetic diet for a child or teenager that is picky about what they eat can be a nightmare. The main focus of a diabetic diet is to get your nutrients and calories from low carb fruits and vegetables. So what do you do if your child refuses to eat these?

Juvenile diabetes is one of the biggest challenges a parent can face, especially if the child is a picky eater. It requires careful meal planning and watching everything your child eats, at home and away. It is not necessarily an easy thing to do, especially with an uncooperative child.

There are, however, some things you can do to get your child on the program for success. These things may seem small, but they add up to big lifestyle changes for your family.

Rewards

Children act based on what is in it for them. Base rewards such as new toys or games or an allowance on how well they stick to their diabetic diet without complaint. This is often enough incentive to get an otherwise uncooperative child to eat their vegetables. Here are some examples of rewards you can offer your child.

- Sugar free dessert if they eat all their dinner

- Time on the video game system after dinner

- A later bedtime

- Allowance money

- Staying over at friend's houses

- Eating out once a month if they follow their diet the rest of the time

Sneaky Substitutions

Make small substitutions in your meal planning that the child is not likely to object to. If you eat a lot of pizza, start making the crust thinner and alter the toppings you put on it. Instead of buying premade pizzas high in carbohydrates, make your own at home from scratch.

You can do the same thing with countless other dishes that are favorites with children. Make a list of all of the foods that your child likes, and search the internet for diabetic recipes for the same foods. The foods will be diabetic friendly in nature, but taste similar to the regular version of the meal. This way your child may absently say, "This tastes a little different tonight," rather than "I'm not eating that!"

It is most important to find substitutions for your child's comfort foods. Comfort foods are important to kids. When they don't get these foods they can actually become angry or depressed. It is important to find substitutes for these foods. Some of the foods you can turn into diabetic diet recipes that kids love include:

- Macaroni and Cheese

- Chicken Nuggets

- Enchiladas

- Sweet potato fries

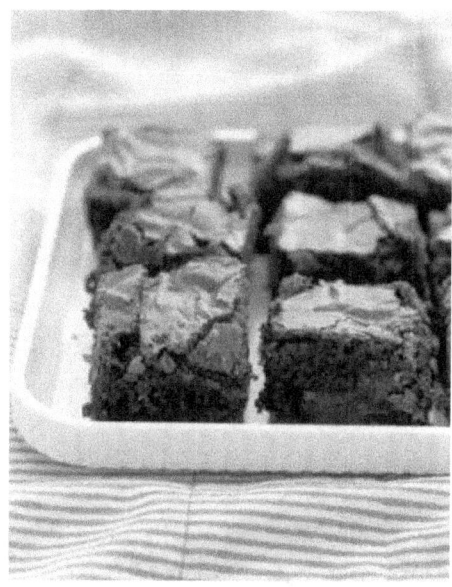

Dessert is a big one for children and teenagers. The prospect of going without dessert can be enough to make a child refuse to eat anything. Look for diabetic dessert recipes for your child's favorite desserts made with sugar substitutes. They probably won't even notice the difference, and the dessert will be a much better reward option than yogurt or fruit. Here are some suggestions.

- Sugar free, gluten free brownies (made with rice flour and sugar substitute)

- Sugar free, low fat cheesecake

- Sugar free chocolate cake

- Sugar free apple pie

- Sugar free ice cream

Spice it Up

Some children just don't like the taste of vegetables. With all of the high carb and calorie foods that we raise our children on today, it is no wonder that they consider vegetables and fruits to be bland and without a good taste. So, spice it up a bit, kick it up a notch, and give them something they can live with.

For example, an easy thing to do is put a little bit of thin cheese sauce over broccoli or mixed vegetables. This gives the vegetables a unique flavor that kids love and enjoy. Another thing you can do is experiment with herbs and spices. Season your vegetables differently each night until you find something your child enjoys. This is made easier by the invention of seasonings such as Mrs. Dash, a brand that has a whole line of different flavors in a bottle that are completely sodium and sugar free.

To get children to eat fruits, you can kick them up a notch by adding the fruit to flavored yogurt. You may also want to try topping fruit with sugar free whipped cream. If you cannot get your child to eat fruits such as apples, try getting some sugar free caramel dipping sauce. Eventually your child will recognize fruits as some of the sweet things they are allowed to have, and they will be more likely to eat them.

Be the Parent

Ultimately, a good diabetic diet contains foods that many children and teenagers would prefer not to eat. Sometimes you will just have to put your foot down and say, no, you are going to eat your dinner. Eventually they will get tired of going hungry and they will eat what is put in front of them.

In short, sometimes you just have to be the parent and tell your child what they are going to do. No, you cannot force feed them. But you can give them both positive and negative incentive to follow along with the diet.

More Tips on Getting Kids to Eat Vegetables

Getting kids to eat something they should be getting the most of throughout their lives is difficult at best. It is even more important for kids with diabetes, because they cannot eat other foods instead to get full. However, you can easily manage to get your kids to eat their vegetables through these tips.

- Take your kids grocery shopping. Allow them to pick out the fruits and vegetables that look good and smell good to them. Give them ideas on how they can be prepared and eaten, and let them make the choice.

- Let your kids into the kitchen with you. Let them see how the vegetables are prepared, and let them help make them. They will be more likely to try something they helped prepare.

- Have a night where the only thing on the plate is vegetables. You can serve up a Portobello mushroom burger with lots of veggies on the side. This means that your child has no choice but eat the vegetables or go hungry, and they are still getting the protein they need from the Portobello. Beans is another example that can be used. This is a great way to get children to try vegetables they have never had before. Once they try them they may discover they like them and will eat them with no problem in the future.

Recommended Daily Allowances for Diabetic Children

When planning a diabetic diet for children and teens, it is important to keep in mind that their bodies are growing. As such, they need more of certain nutrients than adults must have. It is helpful in this case to know the daily allowances that your child should be taking in each day.

- 6-11 servings of grains (a serving being a slice of bread or ½ cup rice)

- 3-5 servings of vegetables

- 2-4 servings of fruits

- 2-3 servings of dairy

- 2-3 servings of protein

Remember that bad fats should be eliminated, as should sweets. However, good fats should still be introduced into the diet for overall health. Cutting out fat completely is a bad idea, especially when it comes to growing kids.

The Difference Between a Diabetic Diet and a Low Glycemic Index Diet

Truthfully, a low glycemic index diet is a type of diet that can be used by diabetics in some cases. However, it differs from a traditional diabetic diet in one important fact. It does not count carbohydrates.

What is a Glycemic Index Diet?

The Glycemic Index of a food is a number assigned to that food based on how quickly the food raises blood sugar levels, and to what extent. The food may be assigned a number as low as fifteen or as high as two hundred. Generally, foods with a glycemic index of sixty or lower are healthy for diabetics.

A glycemic index diet uses this assigned number to determine whether or not a food is healthy to eat. You of course must adhere to serving sizes in order for the glycemic index to work properly. However, the diet itself relies on your ability to look up the glycemic index for foods. It does not count carbohydrates, and does not guarantee that you will not eat too many carbohydrates throughout the day or within one meal.

Why Diabetics Shouldn't Use the Diet

The problem with using the glycemic index to plan a diet for diabetics is that it is not a widely accepted form of diet as of yet. It has really just had its beginnings, and more research is needed. In fact, the glycemic index for most vegetables is entirely unknown.

Because many foods have not had a glycemic index calculated, and because these calculations may vary depending on the source, it is not a very accurate way to plan a diabetic diet. In addition, discovering the glycemic index of foods usually requires a visit to a website, something that may not be possible when you are out and about or at the grocery store. In short, a low glycemic index diet is difficult to follow and may not be the best choice for diabetics.

Who Can Use a Glycemic Index Diet

A low glycemic index diet may be a good option for people who do not have diabetes but have a high risk for the disease. Eating a low glycemic index diet can greatly improve your chances of not getting diabetes, by keeping your blood sugar from spiking and plummeting. However, for more serious individuals and diabetics themselves, it is not a good choice of diet.

Successful Diets for Diabetics

Diabetics are much more likely to have success with a diet that works off of exchanges or that counts carbohydrates, as discussed earlier. These diabetic diets are much easier to manage and maintain because the carbohydrate content of foods is well established and easily determined. It is also highly accurate, because scientific evidence of how carbohydrates raise blood sugar levels is well established.

Conclusion

The diabetes diet is something that must be tailored for each individual. It is not something you can jump into lightly. While prepared diet plans may work for certain individuals, the same diet plan that works for one person may not work for someone else.

It is extremely important that all of your health conditions and concerns are addressed in your diet plan, not just cutting sugars and carbohydrates. Discuss with your doctor in detail the type of diet you need to be on. Diets may vary based on the need to lose weight, pregnancy, nursing mothers, high blood pressure, high cholesterol, high triglycerides, and other health factors. The amount of calories and carbohydrates you need each day or each meal is something very personal to the individual, and therefore should be discussed in depth with a doctor or nutritionist.

However, the information presented here will help you take the information provided by your doctor and nutritionist and put it to use. You will be able to develop and implement your own diabetic diet plan. You will also be able to stick to that plan for your continued good health.

Remember, this is not about creating a short term diet. This is about making lifestyle changes that will stick with you for the rest of your life. The information presented to you in these pages and by your doctor is not meant to be short lived, but is meant to make you change your way of thinking, and eating, for a healthier you.

And, in the end, that is what it is all about. It is about getting healthy, taking as few medications as possible, and managing your blood sugar naturally. With those goals in mind, you should be able to take the information learned here and from other sources to see a successful end to your dieting experience.

www.ingramcontent.com/pod-product-compliance
Lightning Source LLC
Chambersburg PA
CBHW082203290526

45794CB00008B/3406